BASIC FIRST AID POCKET GUIDE

"Be prepared for emergencies: A comprehensive pocket guide to First Aid"

Thomas J. Barron

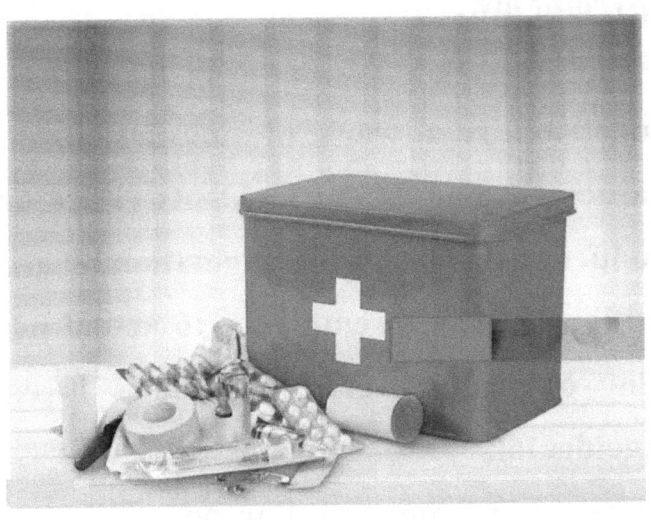

Copyright @ 2024 Thomas J. Barron

All rights reserved. No part of this publication may be reproduced, distributed, or transmitted in any form or by any means, including photocopying, recording, or other electronic or mechanical methods, without the prior written permission of the publisher, except in the case of brief quotations embodied in critical reviews and certain other non-commercial uses permitted by copyright law.

This book is a work of non-fiction. Names, characters, places, and incidents either are the product of the author's imagination or are used fictitiously. Any resemblance to actual persons, living or dead, events, or locales is entirely coincidental.

Published by Thomas J. Barron

TABLE OF CONTENTS

CHAPTER 1 7
Introduction 7
Importance of First Aid 8
Purpose of the Pocket Guide 10
How to Use this Guide 12

CHAPTER 2 15
Basic First Aid 15
Definition 15
Objectives 16
Key Principles 18
Essential Concepts 20

CHAPTER 3 23
Essentials for a First Aid Kit 23
What to Include in a First Aid Kit 23
Where to Keep the First Aid Kit 26

CHAPTER 4 30
Preparing for Common Emergencies 30
Steps to Take in an Emergency Situation 30
Assessing the Situation 32
Prioritizing Care 34
Calling for Help 35

CHAPTER 5 38
Basic First Aid Techniques 38
- Bleeding and Wound Care 38
- Burns 45
- Fractures and Sprains 50
- Insect Bites and Stings 55
- Heat and Cold Emergencies 58
- Choking 68

CHAPTER 6 73
Special Circumstances 73
- First Aid for Children and Infants 73
- First Aid for Elderly Individuals 75
- First Aid for Pets 78

CHAPTER 7 82
Common Medical Emergencies 82
- Heart Attack 82
- Stroke 85
- Allergic Reactions 89
- Seizures 93

CHAPTER 8 97
Tips for Staying Safe 97
- Prevention 97

Basic Safety Measures 100
First Aid Kit Maintenance 103
Educating Others on First Aid 105

CHAPTER 9 109

Conclusion 109

Review 109
Importance of Being Prepared 111
Final Thoughts. 113

CHAPTER 10 BONUS 115

Some sample workout plans for beginners 115

1. Monday: 115
2. Tuesday: 115
3. Wednesday: 116
4. Thursday: 116
5. Friday: 116
6. Saturday: 117
7. Sunday: 117
8. Monday: 117
9. Tuesday: 118
10. Wednesday: 118
11. Thursday: 119
12. Friday: 119
13. Saturday: 120

14. Sunday: 120
15. Monday: 120
16. Tuesday: 121
17. Wednesday: 121
18. Thursday: 122
19. Friday: 122
20. Saturday: 122

CHAPTER 1

Introduction

Mary often goes on long hikes in the woods with her friends. One day, during a hike, her friend falls and twists her ankle. Mary panicked and didn't know what to do as they were deep in the woods with no access to medical assistance.

Fortunately, Mary remembered that she had BASIC FIRST AID POCKET GUIDE in her backpack. She quickly pulled it out and looked up the section on sprained ankles. The guide instructed her to elevate and ice the injured area, as well as wrap it with a bandage. Mary followed the instructions and it helped to reduce her friend's swelling and pain.

The pocket guide also provided additional tips on how to care for the injury until they could get back to civilization. It advised them to take breaks and not put too much weight on the injured ankle, as well as to give her friend some over-the-counter pain medication.

Thanks to the BASIC FIRST AID POCKET GUIDE, Mary was able to handle the situation calmly and effectively. Her friend's ankle healed properly and she was back on her feet in no time.

Mary now always carries the pocket guide with her on her hikes, knowing that it will provide her with the necessary knowledge and guidance in case of any other emergencies.

Importance of First Aid

First-aid pocket guides are essential tools that provide quick and easy access to important information on how to manage common medical emergencies. These guides are designed to be compact and portable, making it convenient for individuals to carry with them at all times. From minor injuries to life-threatening situations, a first aid pocket guide is a valuable resource that can make a significant difference in a person's health and well-being.

One of the main benefits of a first-aid pocket guide is its ability to provide immediate instructions. During an emergency, people may become overwhelmed or panic, making it difficult for them to remember the necessary steps to take. A first aid pocket guide acts as a reference, providing clear and concise instructions that can be followed easily. Even in situations where access to medical professionals may be limited, a first-aid pocket guide can help save lives by providing the necessary guidance.

Another important aspect of a first aid pocket guide is its ability to educate individuals on how to prevent accidents and injuries. These guides often include information on common hazards and provide tips on how to minimize the risk of accidents. By being aware of potential dangers and knowing how to prevent them, people can avoid potential emergencies in the first place.

Moreover, first-aid pocket guides are beneficial for individuals who may not have formal training in first aid. They are designed to be user-friendly, with illustrations and simple language that can be understood by anyone. This makes it possible for individuals who are not medical professionals to provide assistance and potentially save lives in an emergency situation.

First aid pocket guides are also useful for professionals who deal with medical emergencies, such as outdoor enthusiasts, teachers, and caregivers. These guides act as a quick reference guide, providing them with the necessary information to respond to emergencies efficiently and effectively. This is especially important in situations where access to medical help may be hindered, such as during outdoor activities or in remote areas.

In conclusion, the importance of a first aid pocket guide cannot be overstated. These compact and portable guides provide life-saving information, educate individuals on accident prevention, and are useful for both novice and trained first-aiders. It is crucial to have a first aid pocket guide on hand at all times, as you never know when an emergency may occur. With the right knowledge and guidance, a first aid pocket guide can make a significant difference in the outcome of an emergency situation.

Purpose of the Pocket Guide

The purpose of a pocket guide is to provide quick and easy access to important information on a specific topic. In the case of a first-aid pocket guide, its purpose is to provide essential instructions and tips on how to manage common medical emergencies.

A first-aid pocket guide is designed to be compact and portable, making it convenient for individuals to carry with them at all times. Its size and format make it easy to store in a bag, pocket, or car, ensuring that it is always within reach in case of an emergency.

The primary purpose of a first-aid pocket guide is to provide immediate instructions during an emergency. In a high-stress or panic-inducing situation, people may have a hard time trying to remember what steps to take. A first aid pocket guide acts as a reliable source of reference, providing clear and concise instructions that can be followed easily. This can be life-saving in situations where access to medical professionals is limited.

Another purpose of a first-aid pocket guide is to educate individuals on how to prevent accidents and injuries. Most guides include information on common hazards and provide tips on how to minimize the risk of emergencies. By being aware of potential dangers and knowing how to prevent them, people can avoid accidents and injuries in the first place.

Furthermore, a first-aid pocket guide is beneficial for individuals who may not have formal training in first aid. Its user-friendly layout, with illustrations and simple language, makes it easy for anyone to understand and follow. This makes it possible for individuals who are not medical professionals to provide assistance and potentially save lives in emergency situations.

A first-aid pocket guide also serves as a quick reference guide for professionals who deal with medical emergencies, such as outdoor enthusiasts, teachers, and caregivers. Its compact size and organized format provide them with the necessary information to respond to emergencies efficiently and effectively. This is particularly vital in situations where access to medical help may be limited.

In conclusion, the purpose of a first-aid pocket guide is to provide life-saving information, educate on accident prevention, and serve as a quick reference guide for both novices and trained first-aiders. It is an essential tool that should be carried at all times, as it can make a significant difference in the outcome of an emergency situation.

How to Use this Guide

Using the BASIC FIRST AID POCKET GUIDE is simple and straightforward. Here are some tips on how to make the most out of this guide:

1. Familiarize yourself with the layout: This guide is organized into several sections, each covering a

different topic. Take some time to familiarize yourself with the layout so that you can easily find the information you need during an emergency.

2. Always carry it with you: This guide is meant to be compact and portable, so make sure to always have it with you - in your bag, pocket, or car. You never know when an emergency may occur, and having this guide on hand can be lifesaving.

3. Quickly assess the situation: In an emergency, it is crucial to stay calm and quickly assess the situation. Use the guide to determine the type and severity of the injury or illness, and follow the appropriate instructions.

4. Follow the step-by-step instructions: The guide provides step-by-step instructions on how to respond to different medical emergencies. Make sure to follow the steps carefully and sequentially for the best outcome.

5. Do not hesitate to call for professional help: While this guide is useful in providing first aid care, it is not a substitute for professional medical assistance. If the situation is serious or you are unsure of what to do, do not hesitate to call for professional help.

6. Keep learning: A first-aid pocket guide is a valuable resource, but it is essential to remember that it is not a replacement for formal first aid training. Consider taking a first aid course to further improve your skills and knowledge.

By following these tips and using this guide, you can effectively respond to emergencies and provide the necessary care until professional help arrives. Remember to always prioritize safety and follow the guidelines closely for the best outcomes.

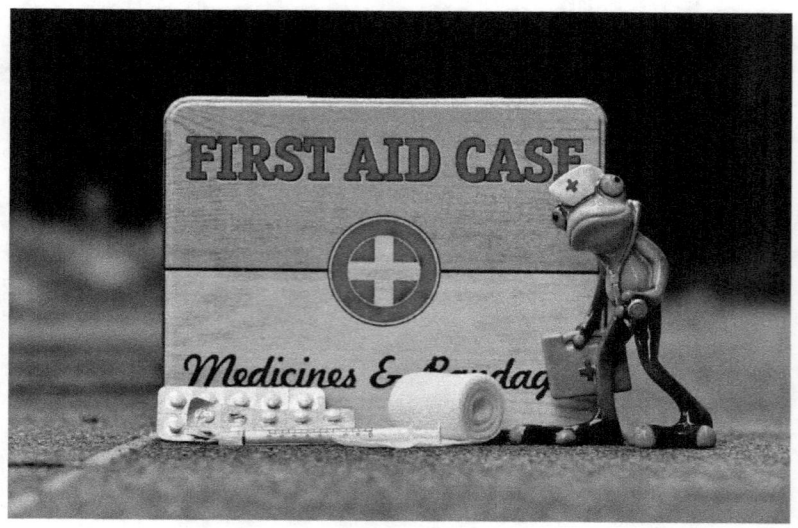

CHAPTER 2
Basic First Aid

Definition

Basic first aid refers to the immediate and initial assistance given to a person who has been injured or has suddenly fallen ill. It involves simple and non-invasive techniques that can be performed by anyone, with or without formal medical training, to help stabilize the person's condition until professional medical assistance is available.

The main focus of basic first aid is to preserve life, prevent further harm, and promote recovery. It includes a wide range of techniques and procedures that can be used to treat various injuries, illnesses, and emergencies.

These may include providing first aid for cuts, burns, fractures, poisoning, choking, asthma attacks, heart attacks, and more.

The purpose of basic first aid is not to provide definitive medical treatment but to stabilize the person's condition until they can receive proper medical care. This is why it is essential to always call for professional help in serious or life-threatening situations. However, in cases where immediate medical assistance is not available, basic first aid can mean the difference between life and death.

In addition to being a life-saving skill, basic first aid also plays a crucial role in promoting safety and preventing accidents. It educates individuals on how to identify, minimize, and respond to potential hazards, reducing the risk of emergencies occurring in the first place.

Overall, basic first aid is a vital skill that everyone should have. It empowers individuals to take immediate action in emergencies, potentially saving lives and preventing further harm. It also promotes a culture of safety, making our homes, schools, workplaces, and communities safer for everyone.

Objectives

The objectives of learning basic first aid are to:

1. Preserve life: The primary objective of basic first aid is to save lives. It equips individuals with the necessary skills to intervene in emergencies and provide immediate assistance that can be critical in stabilizing the person's condition until professional help arrives.

2. Promote recovery: Another objective of basic first aid is to promote the person's recovery and minimize their chances of developing further complications. By providing the appropriate care and following the correct procedures, basic first aid can help support the body's natural healing process.

3. Prevent further harm: Basic first aid also aims to prevent further harm to the person. By following the right steps and using proper techniques, it can help minimize the risk of injuries or illnesses worsening.

4. Provide reassurance: In an emergency, it is crucial to keep the person calm and reassured. Basic first aid skills include communication and interpersonal skills to help the person feel safe and supported.

5. Educate on safety: Basic first aid also has an educational component. It aims to educate individuals on potential hazards and how to prevent accidents from happening. By promoting safety and accident prevention, basic first aid contributes to building a safer society.

6. Build confidence: Knowing how to respond in an emergency can give individuals a sense of empowerment and confidence. Basic first aid training can help individuals feel more prepared and confident in handling potential emergencies.

Overall, the objectives of basic first aid revolve around providing immediate assistance, promoting recovery, preventing harm, and educating on safety. By understanding and achieving these objectives, individuals can become better equipped to handle emergencies and potentially save lives.

Key Principles

The basic principles of first aid are essential guidelines that should be followed in any emergency situation. These principles reflect the fundamental purpose of first aid, which is to preserve life, prevent further harm, and promote recovery.

Here are some of the key principles of basic first aid:

1. Assess the situation: The first step in any emergency is to quickly assess the situation. This involves identifying potential hazards, evaluating the person's condition, and taking necessary safety precautions.

2. Stay calm and act quickly: In a high-stress situation, it is crucial to stay calm and think rationally. Take a deep breath and act quickly, following the necessary steps to provide first aid care.

3. Prioritize safety: The safety of both the injured person and the first aider should be the number one priority in any emergency. Before providing care, make sure the environment is safe, and take necessary precautions to prevent harm.

4. Call for help: In serious or life-threatening situations, always call for professional help as soon as possible. While providing first aid care is crucial, it is not a substitute for proper medical treatment.

5. Follow the correct procedures: Basic first aid procedures are designed to be easy to follow and require no special equipment.

It is important to follow the correct procedures for the best outcome, as improper techniques can cause harm.

6. Communicate effectively: Good communication is essential in emergencies. It is crucial to effectively communicate with the injured person and any bystanders, providing clear instructions and offering reassurance.

7. Continuously assess and monitor: The person's condition should be continuously monitored to see if their condition is improving or worsening. Adjust the first aid care accordingly, and be prepared to provide further assistance if necessary.

By keeping these key principles in mind, individuals can provide effective first aid care and potentially save lives. Basic first aid training can help individuals understand and apply these principles in real-life situations, giving them the knowledge and confidence to act quickly and effectively in an emergency.

Essential Concepts

Basic first aid is an essential skill that everyone should possess. It is the immediate and initial assistance given to a person who has suddenly fallen ill or has been injured. Preserving life, averting additional harm, and fostering recovery are the three main goals of first aid.

There are various concepts and strategies that are essential to understand in basic first aid. These concepts and strategies are crucial for providing effective and safe first aid care. These are a handful of the more significant ones:

1. **Basic Life Support (BLS)**: BLS is the fundamental care given to individuals who have

sustained life-threatening injuries or are in a life-threatening situation. This includes performing CPR, controlling bleeding, and protecting the person's airway.

2. DRABC: An acronym used to remember the sequence of steps to follow in an emergency. It stands for Danger, Response, Airway, Breathing, and Circulation. This helps first aiders gather important information and decide on the necessary actions to take.

3. Primary Survey: The first and most crucial step in any emergency is the primary survey. This involves quickly assessing the person's condition to determine the severity of the injury or illness and identify any potential hazards.

4. Recovery Position: The recovery position is an essential technique used to place an unconscious person in a position that helps maintain an open airway and prevents choking. It also protects the person's airway in case they vomit.

5. RICE: An acronym often used when caring for sports-related injuries. RICE stands for Rest, Ice, Compression, and Elevation and is used to manage soft tissue injuries such as sprains and strains.

6. Secondary Survey: Once the primary survey is completed, a secondary survey is conducted to gather more specific information about the person's condition and look for any other injuries or conditions that may be present.

7. Stop the Bleed: A first aid concept that teaches individuals how to recognize and control life-threatening bleeding. It includes techniques such as applying direct pressure, using a tourniquet, or packing a wound with gauze.

8. Good Samaritan Laws: Laws that provide legal protection to individuals who attempt to provide first aid care during an emergency. These laws encourage bystanders to help in situations where professional medical help is not available.

These are just some of the key concepts and strategies that are crucial to understanding and implementing basic first aid. By familiarizing yourself with these principles and strategies, you can confidently provide first aid care in emergency situations, potentially saving lives.

CHAPTER 3
Essentials for a First Aid Kit

What to Include in a First Aid Kit

A well-stocked first aid kit is an essential item in every household, car, and workplace. Emergencies and accidents can strike at any time, and having a first aid kit readily available can make all the difference in providing quick and effective medical assistance. Whether you are a seasoned outdoorsman or a stay-at-home parent, having a well-prepared first aid kit is crucial. But what should one include in a first aid kit? Here are the essentials for a first aid kit:

1. Basic Supplies:

The first step to creating a first aid kit is to gather basic supplies. This includes adhesive bandages of various sizes, gauze pads, rolls of gauze, adhesive tape, cotton balls and swabs, medical scissors, and tweezers.

These items are the foundation of any first aid kit and are crucial for treating minor cuts, bruises, and scrapes.

2. Medication:

It is essential to include medication in a first aid kit, especially for those with pre-existing medical conditions. This can include pain relievers such as ibuprofen and acetaminophen, antihistamines for allergic reactions, and any prescription medication that may be needed. It is best to keep these medications in their original packaging with clear labeling and expiration dates.

3. Emergency Items:

In case of an emergency, it is essential to have some items in your first aid kit that can help you during critical situations. These items may include a flashlight, batteries, instant cold and hot packs, emergency blanket, and a whistle for signaling for help. These items can come in handy when unexpected emergencies arise, and you are unable to seek immediate medical attention.

4. Personal Protection:

When dealing with injuries and accidents, personal protection is always important.

Some items to include in your first aid kit for personal protection are gloves, face masks, and hand sanitizer. These items not only protect the person administering aid but also help prevent the spread of infections and diseases.

5. First Aid Manual:

Having a first aid manual is essential in a first aid kit. It can provide guidance and instructions for various medical situations. Even if you are well-versed in first aid, having a manual can serve as a useful reference in times of panic and stress.

6. Emergency Contact Information:

In the case of an emergency, it is crucial to have contact information for emergency services as well as your personal healthcare provider. Having this information readily available can save precious time in critical situations.

7. Personalization:

Every person's first aid needs may vary, so it is important to personalize your kit according to your specific needs. For example, if you or a family member has severe allergies, it is important to have an epinephrine auto-injector (EpiPen) in your kit.

If you know how to use specialized equipment such as a tourniquet or splint, it may be wise to include those items as well.

In conclusion, having a well-stocked first aid kit is crucial for handling minor injuries and emergencies. It is important to regularly check and update your kit, replacing expired items and personalizing it to meet your specific needs. By including these essential items in your first aid kit, you can be prepared to handle any minor injury or emergency with confidence and ease.

Where to Keep the First Aid Kit

While having a well-stocked first aid kit is essential, equally important is knowing where to keep it. The location of the first aid kit can make all the difference in terms of its accessibility during an emergency. Here are some places you should consider keeping your first aid kit:

1. Kitchen:

The kitchen is a popular location for a first aid kit in many households. It is often the central gathering place and is easily accessible to everyone.

This makes it an ideal place to store a first aid kit, especially since most accidents, such as burns and cuts, happen in the kitchen.

2. Bathroom:

Another common location for a first aid kit is the bathroom. It is usually the first place people go to when they have a minor injury, making it a convenient location for the kit. However, it is important to keep in mind that bathrooms can be damp and humid, which can affect the shelf life and effectiveness of certain medications and supplies.

3. Living area:

Keeping a first aid kit in the living room or common living area can be beneficial, especially for households with small children or older adults. Children tend to spend more time playing in these areas, increasing the chances of accidents. Similarly, older adults may need easy access to a first aid kit in case of medical emergencies.

4. Workplace:

If you have a job that involves potential hazards, it is important to keep a first aid kit at your workplace. This is especially necessary for those working in construction, factories, or any other physically demanding jobs. Having a first aid kit readily available can help treat minor injuries quickly, reducing the risk of complications.

5. Car:

Accidents can happen at any time, even while traveling. Keeping a first aid kit in your car can be useful in case of minor injuries while on the road. It is also important to have a first aid kit while camping or participating in outdoor activities.

6. Travel:

It is important to have a first aid kit with you while traveling, especially when going to remote or rural areas. The kit can be a lifesaver in case of an emergency when medical help may not be readily available.

7. Visibility:

No matter where you choose to keep your first aid kit, it is important to make sure it is easily visible and accessible to everyone. Placing a bright sticker or label on the box can make it stand out and serve as a reminder to restock and replace supplies regularly.

In conclusion, the location of your first aid kit is crucial in ensuring its accessibility and effectiveness during an emergency. It is important to choose a location that is easily accessible to everyone and can provide a safe and convenient place for the kit. By keeping these factors in mind, you can be better prepared to handle any minor injury or emergency.

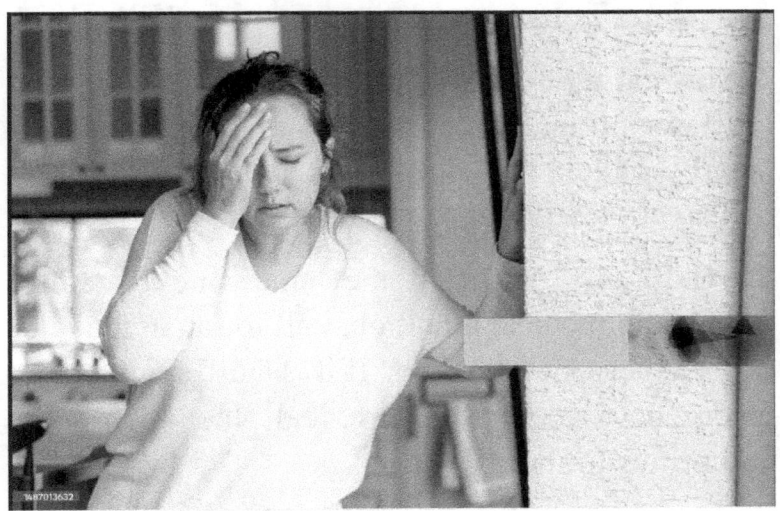

CHAPTER 4
Preparing for Common Emergencies

Steps to Take in an Emergency Situation

1. Stay calm and assess the situation: The first and most important step is to remain calm and think clearly. Take a few deep breaths and try to assess the situation without panicking.

2. Call for help: If the emergency requires immediate medical attention, call for an ambulance or the emergency services. If it is a different type of emergency, such as a fire, call the appropriate authorities for help.

3. Check for any dangers: Before taking any action, make sure that the area is safe or if there are any potential hazards that could endanger you or others. If possible, remove yourself from danger and try to move to a safe location.

4. Follow the emergency procedures: If the emergency is taking place in a public place, there may be specific emergency procedures to follow. Follow these procedures and do not try to be a hero or do something that could put yourself or others in danger.

5. Administer any first aid if necessary: If the situation involves an injury, try to provide basic first aid to the best of your ability. If you are not trained in first aid, keep calm and wait for medical professionals to arrive.

6. Communicate with others: If there are other people around, communicate with them and work together to help resolve the emergency situation. This could involve calling for help, providing first aid, or evacuating the area.

7. Evacuate if necessary: If the situation requires evacuating the area, do so in an orderly and safe manner. Follow any evacuation procedures and help others if needed.

8. Stay informed: If the emergency situation is ongoing, stay informed by listening to updates on the radio, TV, or through other official sources. This will help you make informed decisions and stay safe.

9. Stay put if instructed: In some emergency situations, it may be safer to stay where you are rather than trying to evacuate. If authorities instruct you to stay put, follow their directions and wait for further instructions.

10. Follow up and seek support: After the emergency situation has been resolved, follow up with any necessary actions, such as seeking medical attention or reporting the incident. It is also important to seek emotional support if needed.

Assessing the Situation

1. Take a few moments to calm yourself and assess the situation without panicking. This will help you to think clearly and make rational decisions.

2. Check for any immediate dangers, such as fire, toxic fumes, or a potential for collapse. If there are any immediate threats, remove yourself from danger and move to a safe location.

3. Evaluate the severity of the emergency and whether or not you can handle it on your own or if outside help is needed. This will help you determine your next steps.

4. Determine the best course of action based on the type of emergency.

If it is a medical emergency, the first step should be to call for medical assistance. If it is a natural disaster or other type of emergency, follow the appropriate emergency procedures.

5. If you are in a public place, look for any emergency exit routes or procedures that can guide you out of the building or area safely.

6. Assess the condition of any others who may be involved in the emergency situation. If someone is injured, determine if they require immediate medical attention.

7. Take note of your surroundings and any relevant information that can help emergency responders when they arrive, such as the location of the emergency, any potential hazards, and the number of people involved.

8. If possible, try to communicate with anyone else who may be in the vicinity. Work together to help resolve the emergency situation and provide assistance to anyone who may need it.

9. Stay alert and constantly reassess the situation as it unfolds. The circumstances may change and it is important to adapt your response accordingly.

10. Follow any specific protocols or procedures, such as calling emergency services or following

evacuation routes, to ensure the safety of yourself and others.

Prioritizing Care

1. In a medical emergency, prioritize providing first aid to anyone who may be injured or in need of immediate medical attention.

2. If there are multiple injured parties, assess the severity of their injuries and triage based on the urgency of their condition.

3. Administer first aid to the best of your ability, but do not attempt to provide care beyond your level of training.

4. If the emergency situation involves individuals with pre-existing medical conditions, it is important to prioritize their well-being and provide any necessary care or support.

5. If there are any children, elderly individuals, or people with disabilities present, prioritize their safety and well-being and provide any additional assistance they may need.

6. If anyone requires transportation or other resources to reach medical care, prioritize helping them get to safety and seek necessary assistance.

7. Communicate with emergency responders and provide them with any relevant information or updates on the condition of those affected by the emergency situation.

8. Continue to prioritize the safety and well-being of everyone involved until emergency responders arrive to take over.

9. After the emergency situation has been resolved, prioritize seeking medical attention or emotional support for yourself or anyone else who may need it.

10. Remember to follow up and check in with anyone who may have been affected by the emergency situation, including yourself. This can help with the healing process and ensure that everyone has received the necessary care and support.

Calling for Help

1. If the emergency requires immediate medical attention, call for an ambulance or the appropriate emergency services. Make sure to provide the exact

location of the emergency, the nature of the situation, and any relevant details that can aid the responders.

2. If it is a different type of emergency, such as a fire or natural disaster, call the appropriate authorities for assistance. This may include the fire department, police, or other emergency response teams.

3. Provide clear and concise information to the emergency dispatcher. Speak calmly and slowly, and make sure to listen to any instructions or questions they may have for you.

4. If you are calling from a phone that is not your own, make sure to provide the phone number you are calling from to the emergency dispatcher.

5. If there are multiple people present, ask others to call for help as well. This will help ensure that emergency services are contacted as quickly as possible.

6. Stay on the line with the emergency dispatcher until they tell you it is safe to hang up. They may need to gather more information or provide you with further instructions.

7. If you are unable to call for help, ask someone else to call for you or use a nearby phone or device.

8. After calling for help, stay put if it is safe to do so. If the situation becomes more dangerous, follow any evacuation procedures or seek shelter until help arrives.

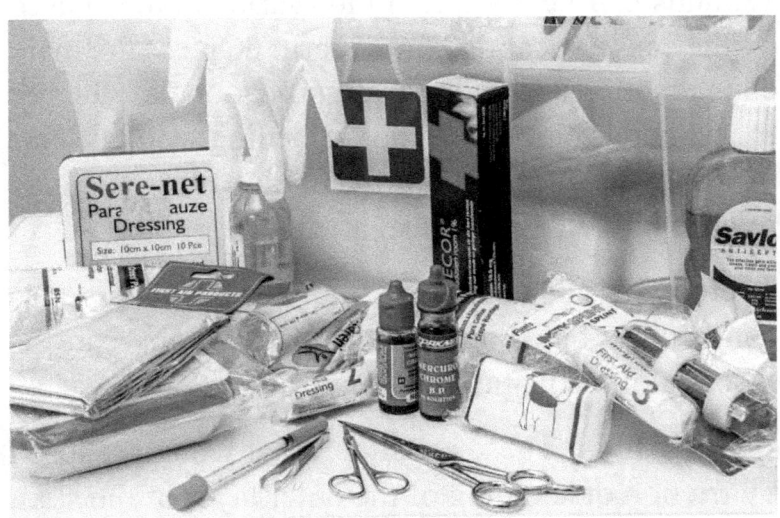

CHAPTER 5
Basic First Aid Techniques

Bleeding and Wound Care

1. Types of Wounds

Wounds can be classified into various types based on the cause, location, and severity. One of the main considerations in wound classification is whether the wound is bleeding or not. Bleeding wounds have the potential to cause significant blood loss and may require immediate medical attention.

Therefore, understanding the types of wounds concerning bleeding and proper wound care is essential in managing these injuries.

1. Abrasions: These are superficial wounds caused by friction or scraping of the outer layer of the skin. While they may bleed, abrasions are usually minor and heal quickly.

They can be treated with soap and water, followed by an antiseptic ointment and a bandage.

2. Lacerations: These are deep cuts or tears in the skin, caused by sharp objects such as a knife or broken glass. Lacerations may bleed heavily and require medical attention to stop the bleeding and prevent infection. The wound should be cleaned with soap and water and controlled with direct pressure using a clean cloth or bandage.

3. Puncture wounds: These are deep, narrow wounds caused by puncturing objects like a needle, nail, or a pointed object. Puncture wounds may bleed, depending on their location and depth. However, the danger lies in the potential for infection, as the wound may seal over and trap bacteria inside. These wounds should be cleaned with soap and water, and if there is any foreign object stuck in the wound, it should be removed before seeking medical attention.

4. Avulsion wounds: These are wounds that result in a loss of tissue or skin, often due to traumatic accidents or severe animal bites. Avulsion wounds can bleed heavily and require prompt medical attention.

The goal of wound care for avulsion wounds is to clean the wound and cover it with a sterile dressing until medical help can be obtained.

5. Gunshot wounds: These are penetrating wounds caused by firearms. Gunshot wounds can cause severe bleeding and may damage internal organs, making them potentially life-threatening.

Immediate medical attention is crucial for gunshot wounds, and wound care should focus on controlling the bleeding and preventing infection.

6. Burns: Burns can result in redness, blistering, and peeling of the skin, depending on their severity. While some burns may not bleed, severe burns can damage blood vessels and cause significant blood loss. Wound care for burns includes cooling the affected area with cold water, covering it with a sterile dressing, and seeking medical help if the burn is extensive or deep.

Proper wound care is essential in promoting healing and preventing complications. In general, the steps for wound care include cleaning the wound with mild soap and water, stopping the bleeding, covering the wound with a sterile dressing, and seeking medical help if necessary. It is crucial to keep the wound clean and dry and change the dressing regularly to promote healing and prevent infection.

In cases of severe bleeding, it is essential to control the bleeding immediately by applying direct pressure. Elevating the injured area above the level of the heart can also help reduce bleeding. If bleeding does not stop with direct pressure, tourniquets may be used as a last resort, but only by trained medical professionals.

In conclusion, understanding the types of wounds concerning bleeding and proper wound care is crucial in managing different types of wounds. While minor wounds can often be treated at home, any wound that involves heavy bleeding, severe pain, or signs of infection should be examined by a medical professional. Prompt and appropriate wound care can significantly aid in the healing process and reduce the risk of complications.

2. Steps to Control Bleeding

1. Apply direct pressure: The first step in controlling bleeding is to apply direct pressure to the wound. This will help to stop or slow down the bleeding by compressing the blood vessels. Use a clean cloth or bandage and apply pressure directly to the wound for several minutes.

2. Elevate the injured area: If the wound is on a limb, it can be helpful to elevate it above the level of the heart. This will reduce blood flow to the injured area and help slow down the bleeding. However, do not elevate the limb if it causes more pain or discomfort.

3. Apply pressure to the pressure points: If the bleeding persists, you can apply pressure to the pressure points in the affected area. These include the brachial artery in the arm and the femoral artery in the leg. Pressing firmly on these areas can help reduce blood flow to the wound and control the bleeding.

4. Use a tourniquet as a last resort: In rare cases of severe bleeding that cannot be controlled with the above methods, a tourniquet may be used as a last resort. A tourniquet involves tightly wrapping a bandage or cloth around the limb above the wound to restrict blood flow. However, this should only be done by trained medical professionals as it can cause further damage if done incorrectly.

5. Seek medical attention: While the bleeding is being controlled, it is important to seek medical attention as soon as possible. This is especially important if the wound is deep, long, or located in a sensitive area. A medical professional will be able to properly clean and dress the wound to prevent infection.

6. Monitor for signs of shock: Severe or prolonged bleeding can lead to shock, which is a life-threatening condition. Watch for signs of shock, such as pale skin, rapid breathing, dizziness, and confusion, and seek immediate medical attention if these symptoms are present.

7. Do not remove any objects stuck in the wound: If the wound is caused by an object such as a knife or a nail, do not attempt to remove it. Removing the object can cause more bleeding and may also cause further damage. Leave this task to a trained medical professional.

In summary, controlling bleeding is essential in wound care to prevent excessive blood loss and promote healing. Following these steps can help effectively control bleeding until medical help can be obtained. Remember to always seek professional help for severe bleeding and closely monitor the wound for signs of infection or other complications.

3. Dressing and Bandaging

In addition to controlling bleeding, dressing and bandaging are important steps in wound care.

Here are some steps to properly dress and bandage a wound:

1. Wash your hands: Before touching the wound, make sure to thoroughly wash your hands with soap and water to reduce the risk of infection.

2. Clean the wound: Using gentle soap and water, clean the wound and surrounding area. If needed, gently remove any debris or dirt from the wound. After giving the wound a thorough rinse, gently dry with a fresh towel.

3. Apply antibiotic ointment: If the wound is clean but not covered in any excess skin, apply an antibiotic ointment to help prevent infection.

4. Choose the appropriate dressing: The type of dressing used will depend on the type and location of the wound. Some options include gauze, adhesive bandages, and adhesive tape. Make sure the dressing is sterile and the appropriate size to cover the wound.

5. Apply the dressing: Carefully place the dressing over the wound, making sure it covers all edges. If the wound is deep, fill it with a sterile gauze before applying the dressing to help absorb any excess fluid.

6. Secure the dressing with bandages: Use adhesive tape, gauze, or bandages to secure the dressing in place. Verify that the bandage is not too tight to permit appropriate blood flow.

7. Change the dressing regularly: It is important to change the dressing regularly, at least once a day or more if the wound is draining heavily. Before changing the dressing, make sure to wash your hands and carefully remove the old dressing.

8. Monitor for signs of infection: Keep an eye on the wound for any signs of infection, such as redness, swelling, or pus. If these symptoms occur, seek medical attention.

9. Seek medical help for large or deep wounds: If the wound is large or deep, it may require medical attention for proper cleaning and dressing. If the wound does not stop bleeding or shows signs of infection, seek medical help immediately.

Properly dressing and bandaging a wound is crucial in promoting healing and preventing infection. Make sure to follow these steps for effective wound care, and seek professional help for any severe or concerning wounds.

Burns

1. Types of Burns

Burns can range from minor injuries, such as sunburns, to more severe injuries that can cause damage to the skin and tissues. The different types of burns require specific wound care approaches for effective healing. Here are the common types of burns and their corresponding wound care:

1. First-degree burns: These are superficial burns that only affect the top layer of the skin. They are typified by pain, moderate swelling, and redness. First-degree burns can be treated at home with cool water, aloe vera, and over-the-counter pain medication. Keep the burn clean and covered with a sterile dressing, and change the dressing regularly.

2. Second-degree burns: These burns involve deeper layers of the skin and are characterized by redness, swelling, and blistering. Second-degree burns can also be treated at home, but it is essential to seek medical attention if the burn is larger than three inches or affects sensitive areas like the face, hands, or feet. Clean the wound daily and apply an antibiotic ointment. Change the dressing regularly and seek medical help if the burn shows signs of infection.

3. Third-degree burns: These are the most severe types of burns and require immediate medical attention. Third-degree burns can cause damage to the deeper layers of the skin, such as nerves, muscles, and bones. Wound care for third-degree burns may involve cleaning the wound, applying antibiotic ointment, and covering it with a sterile dressing. In some cases, skin grafting may be necessary for proper healing.

4. Chemical burns: These burns are caused by contact with strong acids or alkalis. The first step in wound care for chemical burns is to flush the affected area with cool running water for at least 20 minutes. Seek medical help immediately, as these burns can cause severe damage to the skin and tissues.

In summary, different types of burns require specific wound care approaches for proper healing. Proper wound care for burns can help alleviate pain, prevent infection, and promote healing. It is essential to seek medical help for severe burns or if the wound shows signs of infection to prevent further complications.

2. First Aid for Burns

Burn victims must receive first assistance in order to reduce damage and encourage healing. Burns can range from minor injuries to life-threatening emergencies, and proper care should be given immediately.

Here are some important steps to follow in case of a burn:

1. Remove the source of heat:

Taking the heat source out of the burn is the first step in treating it. If the burn was caused by fire, the person should stop, drop, and roll to smother the flames. In case of chemical burns, immediately remove any clothing or jewelry that may have come in contact with the chemical to prevent further injury.

2. Cool the burnt area:

Quickly cool the burnt area with cool running water for at least 10-15 minutes. This helps to reduce pain and swelling and prevents the burn from spreading deeper into the skin. Do not use ice or ice water as it may cause further damage to the skin.

3. Remove any clothing or jewelry:

If clothing or jewelry is stuck to the burnt area, do not try to remove it. Instead, cut around the affected area to safely remove any clothing or jewelry. If any pieces are stuck, leave them in place and seek medical help.

4. Cover the burn:

After cooling the burn, cover it with a sterile gauze or a clean cloth. This protects the affected area from infection and reduces pain. Do not use cotton as it can stick to the burn and cause further damage.

5. Seek medical help:

Serious burns should be assessed and treated by a medical professional. Seek medical help if the burn is larger than three inches, deep, or if it covers major joints such as the hands or feet. Seek immediate medical attention if the burn is on the face, hands, feet, groin, or buttocks.

6. Administer pain relief:

Over-the-counter pain medication like acetaminophen or ibuprofen can help relieve pain and discomfort. Check with a doctor before giving any medication to children.

7. Keep the burn clean:

Keep the burn clean and change the dressing regularly to prevent infection. Wash your hands before and after touching the burn, and avoid popping any blisters that may form.

If the burn blisters on its own, leave the blister intact as it provides a barrier against infection.

8. Watch for signs of infection:

Keep an eye out for any signs of infection such as increased pain, redness, swelling, discharge, or fever. If you notice any of these symptoms, seek medical help right away.

In addition to these steps, it is important to practice good burn prevention techniques. This includes being cautious around hot objects, keeping flammable items away from heat sources, and wearing protective gear when handling chemicals or performing potentially hazardous tasks.

In conclusion, first aid for burns involves removing the source of heat, cooling the burn, covering the affected area, seeking medical help if necessary, administering pain relief, keeping the burn clean, and watching for signs of infection. Remember to seek medical attention for serious burns and practice prevention to avoid future burns.

Fractures and Sprains

1. Types of Fractures and Sprains

Fractures and sprains are common types of injuries that can happen to bones and muscles. They can occur due to various reasons, such as accidents, sports injuries, or falls. While both fractures and sprains involve damage to the musculoskeletal system, there are significant differences between them in terms of causes, symptoms, and treatment.

Fractures are breaks or cracks in bones that can be partial or complete. They can occur due to a sudden force or trauma to the bone, such as a fall, a sports injury, or a car accident. The severity of a fracture depends on the amount of force applied and the strength of the bone. Some common types of fractures include:

1. Simple (closed) fracture: The bone is broken, but the skin is not pierced.

2. Compound (open) fracture: The bone breaks through the skin, causing an open wound.

3. Greenstick fracture: The bone bends and breaks, resembling a green twig.

4. A comminuted fracture is a fractured bone that has numerous broken parts.

5. Stress fracture: Tiny cracks in the bone caused by repetitive stress.

Common symptoms of a fracture include pain, swelling, bruising, and difficulty moving the affected area. In more severe cases, the bone may be visibly misaligned or protrude through the skin. Treatment for fractures depends on the severity and location of the injury. It may include immobilization with a cast or splint, surgery to realign the bone, and rest to allow for proper healing.

Sprains, on the other hand, are injuries to the ligaments that connect bones to each other. They often occur when the ligaments are stretched or torn due to sudden twisting or impact to a joint. Some common types of sprains include:

1. Ankle sprain: The most common type of sprain, usually occurs due to a sudden twist of the ankle.

2. Wrist sprain: Often happens during sports or when falling on an outstretched hand.

3. Knee sprain: Common in athletes and can involve multiple ligaments.

Pain, swelling, bruising, and trouble moving the afflicted joint are signs of a sprain. Depending on the severity of the sprain, treatment may involve rest, ice, compression, and elevation (RICE method), physical therapy, and in severe cases, surgery.

In conclusion, fractures and sprains are both injuries that affect the musculoskeletal system, but differ in terms of causes, symptoms, and treatment. While fractures involve breaks or cracks in bones, sprains involve damage to ligaments in joints. If you experience severe pain or swelling after an injury, it is essential to seek medical attention to determine the best course of treatment and ensure proper healing.

2. First Aid for Fractures and Sprains

In the event of a fracture or sprain, proper first aid is crucial to minimize pain and discomfort, prevent further injury, and promote proper healing. Here are some essential first aid steps to take for these injuries:

1. Stay Calm: In case of an injury, it is essential to stay calm and keep the injured person calm as well. Panicking or moving the affected area too much can worsen the injury.

2. Assess the situation: Before providing any first aid, check the affected area for any visible deformities, swelling, or discoloration. This will help determine the type and severity of the injury.

3. Stop any bleeding: If there is any bleeding from a wound, apply gentle pressure using a clean cloth or bandage to stop it. Avoid moving or manipulating the injury.

4. Immobilize the affected area: To prevent further damage and reduce pain, immobilize the affected area with a splint or brace. This will also help to keep the bone or joint in place and reduce the risk of further injury.

5. Apply cold compress: For swelling and pain, apply a cold compress or ice pack to the affected area. This will lessen discomfort and minimize swelling.

6. Elevate the injured area: Keeping the affected area elevated above the heart can also help reduce swelling and pain.

7. Seek medical help: It is important to seek medical attention, even for seemingly minor fractures or sprains. A healthcare professional can properly assess the injury and provide appropriate treatment.

8. Follow medical advice: After seeking medical help, follow all instructions and recommendations given by healthcare professionals for proper healing. This may include resting, taking medication, or attending physical therapy sessions.

It is essential to note that not all fractures and sprains can be treated with first aid alone. Some may require surgery or specialized medical treatment. In such cases, it is crucial to seek immediate medical attention to prevent further damage and ensure proper healing.

Insect Bites and Stings

1. Types of Insect Bites and Stings

Insect bites and stings can cause discomfort, pain, and even allergic reactions in some cases. They can be caused by a variety of insects, such as mosquitoes, bees, wasps, and ticks. Here are some common types of insect bites and stings and their characteristics:

1. Mosquito bites: These are small, red, itchy bumps that are caused by the bites of female mosquitoes. They can occur anywhere on the body and are most common during warm weather.

2. Bee stings: Bees have a barbed stinger that releases venom into the skin when they sting. The affected area will usually have a red, swollen bump, and may also have a white spot in the center. Bee stings can occasionally result in extremely serious allergic reactions.

3. Wasp stings: Similar to bee stings, wasps have a stinger that releases venom when they sting. The affected area will be red, swollen, and painful, and may also have a white spot in the center.

4. Fire ant bites: These bites typically cause red, itchy bumps that turn into blisters and can become pus-filled over time. Unlike mosquito bites that occur in isolated areas, fire ant bites often appear in clusters.

5. Tick bites: Ticks attach to the skin and feed on blood, and can transmit diseases such as Lyme disease. Tick bites appear as small, red bumps and may have a bullseye-like pattern in certain cases.

6. Flea bites: Flea bites can cause red, itchy bumps that often occur in clusters or lines on the skin. They are commonly found around the ankles and can be transmitted by pets.

7. Spider bites: Most spider bites are harmless and will cause a mild reaction, such as redness and swelling. However, bites from venomous spiders, such as black widows or brown recluses, can cause more severe symptoms and should be treated immediately.

It is important to note that symptoms and reactions to insect bites may vary from person to person. While most insect bites and stings can be treated with home remedies, severe allergic reactions or symptoms should be taken seriously and medical attention should be sought.

2. First Aid for Insect Bites and Stings

While insect bites and stings can be painful and uncomfortable, most can be treated with simple first aid measures at home. Here are some steps to follow:

1. Remove the stinger: If a bee or wasp sting is visible, gently remove the stinger with a blunt object or by scraping it with a fingernail.

Avoid squeezing or pulling out the stinger, as this can release more venom.

2. Clean the affected area: Wash the affected area with soap and water to prevent infection.

3. Apply a cold compress: A cold compress or ice pack can help reduce pain, swelling, and itching.

4. Take an over-the-counter medication: Over-the-counter pain relievers and antihistamines can help alleviate pain and discomfort.

5. Elevate the area: If the bite or sting is on a limb, elevate it above the heart to reduce swelling.

6. Use hydrocortisone cream: If the bite or sting is itchy, applying hydrocortisone cream or calamine lotion can provide relief.

In severe cases, such as anaphylactic shock or severe allergic reactions, it is crucial to seek immediate medical attention. Overall, proper first aid and timely medical intervention can help reduce the discomfort and risks associated with insect bites and stings.

Heat and Cold Emergencies

1. Heat Exhaustion and Heatstroke

Heat exhaustion and heatstroke are two heat-related emergencies that can happen when the body is unable to properly regulate its temperature in hot weather. They are serious conditions that require immediate attention and can be life-threatening if left untreated.

Heat Exhaustion:

Heat exhaustion occurs when the body loses a significant amount of fluids and electrolytes due to excessive sweating. This can cause a person to feel weak, dizzy, and nauseous. Other symptoms of heat exhaustion include:

- Headache

- Rapid heartbeat

- Low blood pressure

- Muscle cramps

- Excessive sweating

- Cool, clammy skin

Heat exhaustion can develop into heatstroke if neglected.

First Aid for Heat Exhaustion:

If you suspect someone is experiencing heat exhaustion, take the following steps:

1. Move them to a cooler and shaded area.

2. Loosen or remove any tight clothing.

3. Provide them with cool water to drink.

4. Use a fan or a small towel soaked in cool water to help cool them down.

5. If possible, have them lie down with their feet elevated.

6. Get medical help if the symptoms worsen or continue.

Heatstroke:

Heatstroke occurs when the body is unable to regulate its temperature, and the core body temperature rises to dangerous levels. This can be triggered by extreme heat or physical exertion in hot weather. Symptoms of heatstroke include:

- High body temperature (usually above 103 degrees Fahrenheit)

- Hot and dry skin

- Rapid and strong pulse

- Headache

- Fatigue and weakness

- Nausea and vomiting

- Confusion and disorientation

- Loss of consciousness

Heatstroke is a medical emergency and requires immediate attention.

First Aid for Heatstroke:

If you suspect someone is experiencing heatstroke, take the following steps:

1. Call for emergency medical help immediately.

2. Move the person to a cooler and shaded area.

3. Remove any excess clothing and apply cool, wet cloths to their skin.

4. Fan the person to promote sweating and cooling.

5. If possible, immerse the person in a tub of cool water.

6. Continue to monitor their vital signs until medical help arrives.

Prevention:

Heat exhaustion and heatstroke can be prevented by following these simple tips:

1. Drink plenty of water and electrolyte-rich fluids to stay hydrated.

2. Wear lightweight, loose-fitting clothing in hot weather.

3. Take frequent breaks in a cool and shaded area if working or exercising in the heat.

4. Avoid being outside during the hottest hours of the day.

5. If you must be outside, use sunscreen and wear a hat to protect against sunburn.

Overall, being aware of the signs and symptoms of heat exhaustion and heatstroke, and taking preventive measures can help avoid these heat-related emergencies. Be mindful of your body's need for hydration and rest, particularly in hot weather, to ensure your well-being and safety.

2. Hypothermia

Hypothermia is a condition where the body's core temperature drops below normal, typically below 95 degrees Fahrenheit. It is a serious cold-related emergency that requires immediate attention, as it can be life-threatening if left untreated.

Causes of Hypothermia:

When the body loses heat more quickly than it can generate it, hypothermia sets in. This may occur for a number of causes, such as:

1. Exposure to cold weather without proper protection.

2. Wearing wet clothing in cold or windy conditions.

3. Submersion in cold water.

4. Staying in a cold indoor environment for an extended period.

Symptoms of Hypothermia:

Depending on how severe the situation is, hypothermia can present with different symptoms. In mild cases, a person may experience shivering, numbness, and tingling in the hands and feet. However, as hypothermia progresses, the body's ability to produce heat decreases, and the person may experience confusion, difficulty speaking, and lack of coordination. Other symptoms of hypothermia include:

- Drowsiness

- Weak pulse

- Slow and shallow breathing

- Loss of consciousness

- Blue skin on the fingers and toes

- Muscle stiffness and rigidity

- Slurred speech

- Pale, cold, and dry skin

First Aid for Hypothermia:

If you encounter someone experiencing symptoms of hypothermia, take the following steps:

1. Move the person to a warm and dry place.

2. Remove any wet clothing and replace it with warm, dry clothes or blankets.

3. If possible, seek immediate medical attention.

4. If the person is conscious, provide them with warm beverages, such as hot tea or soup, and avoid giving them alcohol.

5. Use your body heat to warm the person. If you are in a cold environment, lie next to the person and

cover both your bodies with blankets or sleeping bags.

6. If the person stops breathing, start CPR immediately (if trained) and continue until medical help arrives.

Prevention:

Hypothermia can be prevented by following these tips:

1. Dress appropriately for cold weather by wearing warm and layered clothing.

2. Cover your head and ears with a hat and wear gloves or mittens to protect your hands.

3. Avoid prolonged exposure to cold environments and take breaks in a warm and sheltered area if working or exercising in the cold.

4. If you are planning to spend time in a cold outdoor environment, make sure to bring extra warm and dry clothing, as well as emergency supplies, such as a sleeping bag and emergency blankets.

In conclusion, hypothermia is a serious cold-related emergency that requires immediate attention. Being aware of the signs and symptoms can help prevent this condition and ensure the safety and well-being of yourself and those around you.

3. First Aid for Heat and Cold Emergencies

1. Stay calm and assess the situation: In any emergency, it is important to stay calm and assess the situation. This will help determine the appropriate first aid measures.

2. Move to a safe and comfortable location: If possible, move the person to a safe and sheltered area to protect them from further exposure to heat or cold.

3. Monitor vital signs: Check the person's vital signs, such as breathing and heart rate, to assess their condition and determine the severity of the emergency.

4. Call for medical help: If the person is experiencing severe symptoms or is unresponsive, call for emergency medical assistance immediately.

5. Remove excess clothing: In cases of heat exhaustion or heatstroke, remove any tight or excess clothing to help cool down the body.

6. Provide water or fluids: In hot weather, it is crucial to stay hydrated. Provide the person with water or electrolyte-rich fluids to drink to replenish lost fluids.

7. Use cooling methods: Use fans, cool towels, or a cold compress to help cool down the body in cases of heat exhaustion or heatstroke.

8. Use heat sources: If someone is experiencing hypothermia, use body heat or heat packs to warm them up. Avoid using direct heat, such as hot water or heating pads, as it can cause burns.

9. Seek shelter: In cases of cold weather emergencies, seek shelter and use blankets or warm clothing to cover up and protect the body from further cold exposure.

10. Monitor the person's condition: Continue to monitor the person's condition and vital signs until medical help arrives.

11. Follow medical advice: After seeking medical attention, follow all instructions and recommendations given by healthcare professionals for proper treatment and recovery.

12. Prevention is key: To prevent heat and cold emergencies, it is important to be aware of weather conditions and dress appropriately, stay hydrated, and take breaks in a cool or warm environment when exposed to extreme temperatures. Also, knowing how to recognize the signs and symptoms of these emergencies can help prevent them from becoming life-threatening.

Choking

1. Signs and Symptoms

Choking occurs when an object or food becomes lodged in the airway, blocking the flow of air and causing breathing difficulties. This can be a life-threatening emergency that requires immediate action. Knowing the signs and symptoms of choking can help you identify and respond quickly in case of an emergency.

Signs and Symptoms:

1. Difficulty breathing: One of the most common signs of choking is difficulty breathing or gasping for air.

2. Inability to speak or cry: If someone is choking, they may not be able to speak or make noise.

3. Clutching the throat: The person may grasp their throat with their hands, indicating that they are having difficulty breathing.

4. Coughing or gagging: In an attempt to expel the object, the person may cough or gag.

5. Wheezing or noisy breathing: A blocked airway can cause wheezing or noisy breathing sounds.

6. Skin discoloration: The person's skin may turn blue or red due to lack of oxygen.

7. Inability to make sounds: As the airway becomes more blocked, the person may become silent and unable to make any sounds.

8. Loss of consciousness: Without immediate intervention, choking can lead to loss of consciousness and eventually death.

9. Panic or distress: The person may also exhibit signs of distress or panic, such as grabbing at their throat or making frantic gestures.

10. Weak or ineffective cough: If a person has a weak or ineffective cough, it may indicate that their airway is partially blocked.

It is important to note that these signs and symptoms may vary depending on the age and size of the person, as well as the severity and location of the blockage.

Treatment:

If someone is choking and is able to cough or make sounds, encourage them to continue coughing and try to clear the obstruction themselves. However, if the person is unable to cough or speak, or if they are losing consciousness, you must take immediate action and perform the Heimlich maneuver.

This involves standing behind the person and pressing firmly on their abdomen, just below the ribcage, in an upward motion. This can help dislodge the object and clear the airway. If the person becomes unconscious, perform CPR until medical help arrives.

Prevention:

To prevent choking, it is important to:

1. Cut food into small pieces: When feeding young children or elderly adults, cut food into small, bite-sized pieces to prevent choking.

2. Chew food thoroughly: Encourage children and adults to chew their food properly before swallowing.

3. Avoid talking or laughing while eating: Talking or laughing while eating can increase the risk of choking.

4. Avoid giving small objects to children: Keep small objects, such as coins, beads, and marbles, away from children, as they can be potential choking hazards.

5. Know how to respond in an emergency: Knowing how to perform the Heimlich maneuver and CPR can save a person's life in case of choking. Consider taking a first aid or CPR class to learn these vital skills.

In conclusion, recognizing the signs and symptoms of choking and knowing how to respond in an emergency can help prevent a potentially life-threatening situation. Stay vigilant and take necessary precautions to keep yourself and those around you safe from choking hazards.

2. First Aid for Choking

1. Perform the Heimlich maneuver: Stand behind the person and put your arms around their waist. Make a fist with one hand and place it just above the person's belly button, with your thumb towards their abdomen. Then, grasp your fist with your other hand and give quick upward thrusts until the object is dislodged.

2. Use back blows: If the person is unable to stand or if you are unable to perform the Heimlich maneuver, use back blows. Have the person lean forward and using the heel of your hand, give five sharp blows between the shoulder blades.

3. Check for a tongue obstruction: If the person is unconscious and not breathing, open their mouth and check for any visible obstructions. Try using your fingertips to delete whatever you see.

4. Do CPR: As soon as the person loses consciousness, start CPR. Check for a pulse and if no pulse is present, start chest compressions and rescue breaths. Continue CPR until medical help arrives.

5. Seek medical help: Even if the object is dislodged, it is important to seek medical help and get the person evaluated for any potential injuries or complications.

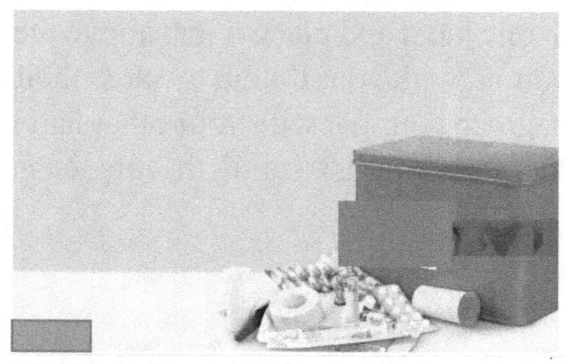

CHAPTER 6

Special Circumstances

First Aid for Children and Infants

1. Choking:

Children and infants have smaller airways and are at a higher risk of choking. If a child or infant is choking, follow the steps for choking first aid listed above, but keep in mind their smaller size.

For infants, use two fingers to perform the Heimlich maneuver, and for children, adjust the strength of your thrusts accordingly. In addition, infants and children may not be able to communicate their symptoms, so be vigilant for signs of distress and take immediate action.

2. Allergic reactions:

Children and infants may be at risk for allergic reactions to foods, insect bites, or other allergens. If a child or infant is having an allergic reaction, it is important to administer an epinephrine auto-injector (e.g. Epi-pen) if available, and call for medical help immediately. If there is no epinephrine available, closely monitor the child's breathing and any changes in their condition.

If their condition worsens, call for emergency help and perform CPR if necessary.

3. Burns:

Young children and infants have delicate skin that can be easily burned. In case of a burn, first remove the child or infant from the source of the burn and cool the affected area with cool (not cold) water for at least 10 minutes. Do not apply ice or butter to the burn. For severe burns, cover the area loosely with a clean, dry cloth and seek medical help.

4. Febrile seizures:

Febrile seizures, which are seizures caused by high fever, are more common in children under the age of 5. If a child has a febrile seizure, lay them on their side and clear the area around them to prevent injury. Do not try to stop the seizure, but instead, focus on ensuring the child's safety and call for emergency help. Afterwards, monitor the child's temperature and seek medical advice.

5. Head injuries:

Children and infants are at a higher risk for head injuries due to their increased activity levels. If a child or infant has a head injury, apply a cold compress to the affected area to reduce swelling.

Monitor the child for any changes in behavior or symptoms, such as loss of consciousness or vomiting, and seek medical help if necessary.

6. Drowning:

Children and infants can drown in as little as 1 inch of water. If a child or infant is found unresponsive in water, immediately remove them from the water and begin CPR if they are not breathing. Call for emergency help and continue CPR until medical help arrives.

It is important to always keep a first aid kit on hand, especially when caring for children and infants. In special circumstances, it is crucial to stay calm and act quickly to provide the necessary first aid. If in doubt, always seek medical help and call for emergency assistance.

First Aid for Elderly Individuals

As we age, our bodies become more susceptible to injuries and medical emergencies. Elderly individuals may also have underlying health conditions that can complicate first aid procedures in case of an emergency.

Knowing how to provide first aid for elderly individuals in special circumstances is important for their well-being. Here are some tips to keep in mind.

1. Falls:

One of the most frequent ways that older people become hurt is from falls. If an elderly person falls, it is important to assess their condition and any visible injuries. If the person is conscious and not injured, help them to a sitting or standing position. If they are injured, do not move them and call for medical help. Use a clean cloth to apply pressure to the wound if there is any bleeding.

2. Stroke:

Strokes are more common in the elderly, and it is important to act quickly if one occurs. If an elderly person is showing signs of a stroke, such as facial drooping, difficulty speaking, or weakness on one side of the body, call for emergency help immediately. While waiting for help to arrive, keep the person comfortable and monitor their condition.

3. Heart attack:

Elderly individuals are also at a higher risk for heart attacks. If an elderly person is showing signs of a heart attack, such as chest pain, difficulty breathing, or dizziness, call for emergency help immediately. Press a clean cloth against the cut if there is any bleeding. If they are conscious, have them take their prescribed medication for a heart attack, such as aspirin.

4. Bleeding:

Elderly individuals may be taking medications that can increase their risk of bleeding. If an elderly person is bleeding, apply pressure to the wound with a clean cloth. If the bleeding does not stop, call for medical help immediately. Also, keep in mind that elderly individuals may be taking blood thinners, so the bleeding may take longer to stop.

5. Choking:

As we age, our ability to chew and swallow may decrease, putting elderly individuals at a higher risk for choking. If an elderly person is choking, perform the Heimlich maneuver carefully, as their bodies may be more fragile. If the person is unconscious, perform CPR until medical help arrives.

6. Medication overdose:

Elderly individuals may have multiple health conditions and take several medications, increasing their risk for medication overdose.

If an elderly person is showing signs of a medication overdose, such as confusion, drowsiness, or difficulty breathing, call for emergency help immediately. If possible, gather the person's medication list to provide to the medical professionals.

7. Burns:

Elderly individuals may have thinner, more delicate skin that can be easily burned. If an elderly person has a burn, immediately remove the person from the source of the burn. Run cool water over the affected area for at least 10 minutes and do not apply ice or butter. Cover the burn loosely with a clean, dry cloth and seek medical help if necessary.

It is important to be prepared and have a first aid kit on hand when caring for elderly individuals. Keep in mind that their bodies may be more fragile and have underlying health conditions that can complicate first aid procedures. If in doubt, always seek medical help and call for emergency assistance.

First Aid for Pets

Our furry friends are an important part of our families, and it is important to know how to provide first aid to them in case of an emergency. In special circumstances, such as during natural disasters or accidents, pets may require immediate medical attention.

Here are some tips for providing first aid to pets on special circumstances.

1. Bleeding:

Pets may get into accidents that can cause bleeding, and it is important to act quickly to stop the bleeding. Apply pressure to the wound with a clean cloth or gauze pad. If the bleeding does not stop, seek veterinary help immediately. In case of severe bleeding, you can apply a tourniquet between the wound and the heart, but this should only be done as a last resort.

2. Burns:

Pets can also get burned from hot objects, chemicals, or fire. If your pet has a burn, immediately remove them from the source of the burn and run cool water over the affected area for at least 10 minutes. Do not apply ice or butter to the burn. Cover the burn loosely with a clean cloth or gauze pad and seek veterinary help if necessary.

3. Insect bites and stings:

Bees, wasps, and other insects can pose a threat to our pets. If you notice your pet has been bitten or stung, remove the stinger if visible and clean the area with soap and water. Apply a cold compress to reduce swelling and seek veterinary help if your pet is showing signs of an allergic reaction, such as difficulty breathing or excessive swelling.

4. Heatstroke:

Pets can suffer from heatstroke, especially in hot weather or if they are left in a car. If your pet is showing signs of heatstroke, such as excessive panting, drooling, or weakness, move them to a cool area and apply cool (not cold) water to their fur. Do not use ice as it can cause the body temperature to drop too quickly. Seek veterinary help immediately.

5. Cuts and wounds:

Just like humans, pets can also suffer from cuts and wounds. If your pet has a cut or wound, clean the area with saline solution or mild soap and water. Apply a clean bandage or gauze pad over the wound, and change it regularly to prevent infection. Seek veterinary help if the wound is deep or does not heal within a few days.

6. Poisoning:

Pets are curious creatures and may ingest toxic substances. If you suspect your pet has been poisoned, call your veterinarian or animal poison control immediately. Unless a medical professional instructs you to do so, avoid forcing vomiting.

7. Transportation accidents:

In case of a transportation accident, such as a car crash, keep your pet calm and check for injuries. If your pet has been injured, seek veterinary help immediately. Make sure to safely secure your pet in a carrier or with a leash to prevent them from running away or causing further injury.

It is important to have a pet first aid kit on hand, especially when traveling with your pet. Keep your veterinarian's contact information handy, and always seek professional help in case of emergencies. Remember to remain calm and act quickly to provide the necessary first aid for your furry friend.

CHAPTER 7

Common Medical Emergencies

Heart Attack

A heart attack, also known as a myocardial infarction, is a medical emergency that occurs when there is a blockage of blood flow to the heart. This can lead to permanent damage to the heart muscle if not treated promptly. Knowing how to recognize and respond to a heart attack is critical for basic first aid knowledge. Here is a guide to understanding and managing a heart attack as a common medical emergency.

Recognizing the Signs and Symptoms

A heart attack can present with a variety of signs and symptoms, but some of the most common ones include:

- Pain or discomfort in the middle of the chest, which can feel like pressure, squeezing, fullness, or another emotion

- Pain or discomfort in the back, neck, jaw, arms, or stomach, among other upper body parts

- Shortness of breath

- Nausea and vomiting

- Cold sweat

- Dizziness or light headedness

- Fatigue

- Trouble speaking

- Anxiety

- Pale or gray skin color

However, not everyone experiencing a heart attack will have all of these symptoms. Some may only experience mild discomfort or no symptoms at all. If you think you may be having a heart attack, you should definitely pay attention to any strange symptoms and get medical assistance right once.

First Aid for a Heart Attack

If you suspect that someone is having a heart attack, follow these steps:

1. Call 911: Call for emergency medical assistance immediately. Time is of the essence when it comes to treating a heart attack, and every minute counts.

2. Help the person to rest: Have them sit down and rest in a position that is comfortable for them. If they are having trouble breathing, allow them to sit in a position that makes it easier for them to breathe, such as propped up with pillows.

3. Loosen any tight clothing: This will help to improve blood flow and ease the person's discomfort.

4. Give them medication if they have it: If the person has been prescribed medication for chest pain, such as nitroglycerin, help them take it as directed.

5. Stay with them: Reassure the person and stay with them until medical help arrives. If they lose consciousness, check for breathing and heartbeat and be prepared to administer CPR if necessary.

Preventing a Heart Attack

While not all heart attacks can be prevented, there are some steps you can take to reduce your risk:

- **Maintain a healthy diet:** Eat plenty of fruits, vegetables, whole grains, and lean proteins to keep your heart healthy.

- **Stay physically active:** Regular exercise can help improve your cardiovascular health.

- **Quit smoking:** Smoking is a significant risk factor for heart disease and can increase your chances of having a heart attack.

- **Control your blood pressure and cholesterol levels:** High blood pressure and cholesterol levels can damage your blood vessels and increase your risk of a heart attack.

- **Manage your stress levels:** Chronic stress can contribute to heart disease. Seek out stress-reduction techniques that are good for you, such as physical activity, meditation, or counseling.

In summary, a heart attack is a medical emergency that requires immediate attention. Knowing the signs and symptoms and how to respond can help save a life. By taking preventive measures, you can also reduce your risk of a heart attack. Remember to always seek medical assistance when needed, and don't hesitate to call for help in an emergency.

Stroke

If you think you may be having a heart attack, you should definitely pay attention to any strange symptoms and get medical assistance right once.

This can lead to permanent brain damage or death if not treated promptly. Knowing how to recognize and respond to a stroke is crucial for basic first aid knowledge. Here is a guide to understanding and managing a stroke as a common medical emergency.

Recognizing the Signs and Symptoms

A stroke can present with a variety of signs and symptoms, but the most common ones include:

- Abrupt numbness or weakness in the arm, leg, or face, often on one side of the body

- Difficulty speaking or understanding others

- Confusion, trouble with vision, or dizziness

- An abrupt, intense headache without a known cause

- Having trouble walking or becoming uncoordinated

- Facial drooping or a lopsided smile

It is essential to act quickly and seek medical help immediately if you suspect someone is having a stroke. The acronym "FAST" can help you remember the signs of stroke:

- Face – ask the person to smile and see if one side of their face droops.

- Arms: Have them extend both arms, and watch to see if one sags down.

- Speech – ask the person to repeat a simple phrase and see if their speech is slurred or strange.

- Time – call for emergency medical assistance immediately if you notice any of these signs.

First Aid for a Stroke

Take these actions if you think someone is having a stroke:

1. Call 911: Time is of the essence when it comes to treating a stroke. Call for emergency medical assistance immediately.

2. Help the person to rest: Have them lie down in a position that is comfortable for them with their head slightly elevated.

3. Note the time: It is important to take note of when the symptoms first started, as this can help medical professionals determine the best course of treatment.

4. Loosen any tight clothing: This will help to improve blood flow and ease the person's discomfort.

5. Keep them calm: Reassure the person and try to keep them calm while waiting for medical help to arrive.

Preventing a Stroke

While not all strokes can be prevented, there are things you can do to lower your risk:

- **Maintain a healthy diet:** Eat plenty of fruits, vegetables, whole grains, and lean proteins to keep your blood pressure and cholesterol levels in check.

- **Stay physically active:** Regular exercise can help improve your cardiovascular health and lower your risk of stroke.

- **Quit smoking:** Smoking is a significant risk factor for stroke and can increase your chances of having a stroke.

- **Keep your blood pressure and cholesterol levels in check:** High blood pressure and cholesterol levels can increase your risk of stroke.

- **Manage your stress levels:** High levels of stress can contribute to stroke.

Look for healthy strategies to deal with stress, like working out, practicing meditation, or seeing a therapist.

In summary, a stroke is a medical emergency that requires immediate attention. Knowing the signs and symptoms and how to respond can help save a life. By taking preventive measures, you can also reduce your risk of a stroke. Remember to always seek medical assistance when needed, and don't hesitate to call for help in an emergency.

Allergic Reactions

An allergic reaction is a medical emergency that occurs when the immune system overreacts to a substance that is otherwise harmless.

These reactions can range from mild to life-threatening and require prompt treatment to prevent serious complications. Knowing how to recognize and respond to an allergic reaction is essential for basic first aid knowledge.

Here is a guide to understanding and managing allergic reactions as a common medical emergency.

Recognizing the Signs and Symptoms

An allergic reaction can present with a variety of signs and symptoms, but some of the most common ones include:

- Itchy, red, or swollen skin

- Hives or welts

- Face, lip, tongue, or throat swelling

- Trouble breathing

- Wheezing or coughing

- Runny or stuffy nose

- Nausea and vomiting

- Diarrhea

- Dizziness or lightheadedness

- Loss of consciousness

These symptoms can occur within minutes of coming into contact with the allergen or up to several hours later. It is essential to pay attention to any unusual symptoms and seek medical help immediately if you suspect an allergic reaction.

First Aid for Allergic Reactions

If someone is experiencing a severe allergic reaction, also known as anaphylaxis, follow these steps:

1. Call 911: Anaphylaxis is a life-threatening medical emergency that requires immediate medical assistance.

2. Give them medication if they have it: If the person has been prescribed an epinephrine auto-injector, such as an EpiPen, help them use it as directed.

3. Help the person to rest: Have them lie down in a position that is comfortable for them with their legs elevated.

4. Note the time: It is essential to take note of when the symptoms first started, as this can help medical professionals determine the best course of treatment.

5. Keep them calm: Reassure the person and try to keep them calm while waiting for medical help to arrive.

Preventing Allergic Reactions

Remaining away from recognized allergens is the best defense against an allergic reaction. Here are some tips to help prevent allergic reactions:

- **Know your allergens:** Be aware of what substances trigger an allergic reaction for you.

- **Read labels:** Always read the ingredients list on product labels to avoid potential allergens.

- **Carry medication:** If you have a known allergen, make sure to carry your prescribed medication, such as an epinephrine auto-injector.

- **Inform others:** Let your family, friends, and coworkers know about your allergies and how to help in case of an allergic reaction.

In summary, an allergic reaction is a medical emergency that requires immediate attention, especially if it is severe. Knowing the signs and symptoms and how to respond can help save a life. By taking preventive measures and being prepared, you can also reduce your risk of experiencing an allergic reaction.

Always seek medical assistance when needed and don't hesitate to call for help in an emergency.

Seizures

A seizure, also known as a convulsion, is a sudden, uncontrolled electrical disturbance in the brain that can cause changes in behavior, movements, or consciousness. Seizures can range from mild to severe and often occur without warning. Knowing how to recognize and respond to a seizure is critical for basic first aid knowledge. Here is a guide to understanding and managing seizures as a common medical emergency.

Recognizing the Signs and Symptoms

The signs and symptoms of a seizure can vary depending on the type of seizure and the individual. Some common signs and symptoms include:

- Loss of consciousness

- Involuntary movements, such as jerking of the limbs

- Staring or repetitive movements

- Difficulty speaking or understanding others

- Confusion or disorientation

- Loss of bladder control

- Headache or fatigue after the seizure

If you witness someone experiencing a seizure, it is essential to stay calm and take note of the duration, type of movements, and any other symptoms that may occur.

First Aid for Seizures

To assist someone experiencing a seizure, do the following:

1. Stay calm: It is important to remain calm and reassuring during a seizure. Do not try to hold the person down or stop their movements.

2. Protect the person from injury: Move any objects out of the person's way to prevent them from hitting or bumping into them. You can also place a soft object, such as a pillow, under their head to prevent injury.

3. Time the seizure: Note the time the seizure starts and ends. If the seizure lasts for more than five minutes, call 911.

4. Turn the person on their side: This will help prevent choking if they vomit or have excess saliva.

5. Stay with the person: Reassure the person and stay with them until the seizure stops or medical help arrives.

Preventing Seizures

While not all seizures can be prevented, there are things you can do to lower your risk:

- **Get enough sleep:** Lack of sleep can trigger seizures in some individuals. Try to get between seven and nine hours each night.

- **Take medication as prescribed:** If you have been prescribed medication for a medical condition that increases your risk of seizures, make sure to take it as directed by your doctor.

- **Avoid known triggers:** Some common triggers for seizures include stress, alcohol consumption, specific foods, or flashing lights. Recognize and attempt to avoid your triggers.

- **Seek treatment for underlying conditions:** Treating underlying conditions, such as epilepsy, brain injury, or stroke, can help reduce the risk of seizures.

In summary, seizures are a common medical emergency that can occur without warning. Knowing the signs and symptoms and how to respond can help save a life.

By taking preventive measures and seeking treatment for underlying conditions, you can also reduce your risk of experiencing a seizure. Remember to always seek medical assistance when needed and don't hesitate to call for help in an emergency.

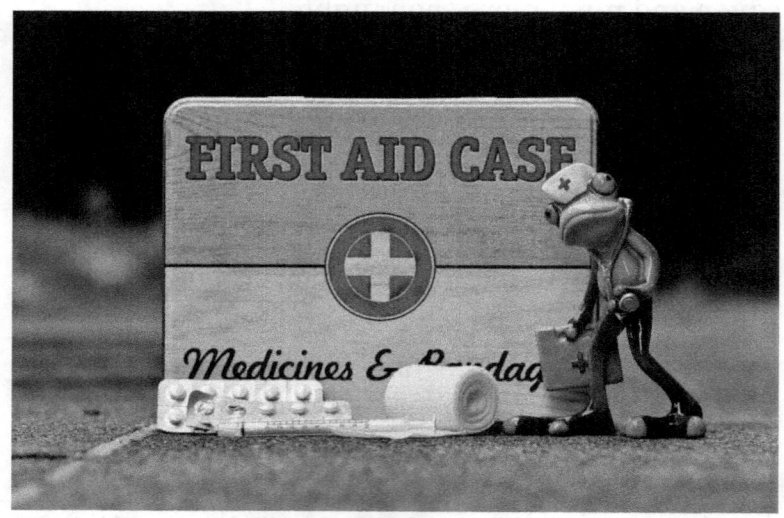

CHAPTER 8

Tips for Staying Safe

Prevention

Prevention is always better than cure, and this is especially true when it comes to staying safe. The world can be a dangerous place, and it's important to be proactive in protecting ourselves. Here are some tips for staying safe and preventing potential risks.

1. Be aware of your surroundings: The first step to staying safe is to be aware of your surroundings at all times. This means paying attention to the people and places around you. Avoid walking alone in areas that are poorly lit or unfamiliar to you. Stay in well-populated areas and always trust your instincts if something feels off.

2. Have a plan: Whether you are going out for the night or taking a trip, it's important to have a plan in place. Make sure someone knows where you are going and when you expect to return. It's also a good idea to have a backup plan in case anything goes wrong.

3. Utilize technology: In today's digital age, there are many apps and devices available that can keep us safe. For example, there are safety apps that allow you to share your location with trusted contacts, and there are wearable devices that can alert authorities in case of an emergency. Utilizing these tools can provide an extra layer of protection.

4. Practice caution with strangers: It's important to remember that not everyone has good intentions. Be cautious when interacting with strangers, especially if they are offering you something or asking for personal information. It's okay to say no and trust your gut if something doesn't feel right.

5. Learn self-defense techniques: Taking a self-defense class can give you the skills and confidence to protect yourself in dangerous situations. Knowing how to defend yourself can be invaluable in case of an attack.

6. Secure your home: Your home should be a safe haven, so take the necessary steps to keep it secure. This includes locking all doors and windows, installing a security system, and using motion-sensor lights. It's also important to keep your personal information, such as your address, private.

7. Be responsible with social media: It's all too easy to overshare personal information on social media, which can make you a target for thieves or predators. Be cautious about what you post online and consider adjusting your privacy settings to limit who can see your posts.

8. Educate yourself on potential risks: Whether it's travel safety, online scams, or natural disasters, it's important to educate yourself on potential risks. Knowing what to expect and how to handle different situations can help you stay safe and avoid dangerous situations.

9. Have an emergency kit: It's always a good idea to have an emergency kit on hand in case of unforeseen events. This may include items like a first-aid kit, non-perishable food, water, and a flashlight. It's better to be prepared than caught off guard.

10. Trust your instincts: Lastly, it's crucial to trust your instincts. If you feel uncomfortable or unsafe, remove yourself from the situation immediately. Don't downplay your gut feelings - they are there for a reason.

In conclusion, staying safe requires a proactive approach and taking necessary precautions. By being aware of your surroundings, having a plan, utilizing technology, and being cautious, you can reduce the risks of potential harm.

Remember to always prioritize your safety and trust your instincts. Stay safe, and stay vigilant.

Basic Safety Measures

Staying safe should be a top priority for everyone, no matter where you are or what you're doing. While it's impossible to completely eliminate all risks, there are basic safety measures that you can take to protect yourself and others. Here are some simple tips for staying safe:

1. Wear a seatbelt: Whether you're driving or in a car as a passenger, wearing a seatbelt is one of the easiest and most effective safety measures you can take. It significantly reduces the risk of serious injury or death in a car accident.

2. Avoid distracted driving: It's no secret that distracted driving is dangerous, yet many people still engage in it. Texting, talking on the phone, eating, or any other activity that takes your focus away from the road can have serious consequences.

Stay safe by keeping your eyes on the road and your hands on the wheel.

3. Practice fire safety: Fires can happen quickly and unexpectedly, so it's important to have basic fire safety measures in place. This includes having working smoke detectors, creating an escape plan, and knowing how to use a fire extinguisher.

4. Use caution with chemicals: Whether at home or work, chemicals can be hazardous. Always read labels and follow instructions for handling and storing chemicals. If you're doubtful, consult a specialist.

5. Be aware of your surroundings when walking: Walking may seem like a simple activity, but it's important to be aware of your surroundings for safety. This includes watching out for potential hazards like uneven sidewalks, staying alert for vehicles or bicycles, and avoiding poorly lit areas.

6. Keep your personal information secure: Identity theft and fraud are becoming increasingly common, so it's important to keep your personal information secure. Be cautious when sharing personal information online, and shred any documents that contain sensitive information.

7. Practice safe food handling: Foodborne illnesses can easily be prevented by following safe food handling practices. This includes washing your hands before handling food, properly storing and refrigerating leftovers, and cooking food to the recommended internal temperature.

8. Use safety equipment: Whether it's a bike helmet, safety goggles, or earplugs, make sure to use the necessary safety equipment for different activities. They can significantly lower the chance of harm.

9. Avoid dangerous activities while under the influence: Whether it's drugs or alcohol, engaging in dangerous activities while under the influence greatly increases the risk of accidents and injuries. Always avoid driving or performing any other potentially dangerous activity while under the influence.

10. Educate yourself and others: It's important to stay informed about safety measures and to educate others on their importance. This can include teaching children about safety, sharing safety tips with friends and family, and staying up-to-date on current safety guidelines and regulations.

By following these basic safety measures, you can greatly reduce the risks of accidents and keep yourself and those around you safe. Remember to always prioritize safety, and stay vigilant.

First Aid Kit Maintenance

Having a well-stocked and properly maintained first aid kit is an essential part of staying safe in any situation. In case of an emergency or injury, a first aid kit can provide the necessary tools and supplies to help until professional help arrives. Here are some tips for maintaining your first aid kit and ensuring it is ready for use at all times:

1. Check expiration dates: Just like with any other medication or product, the items in your first aid kit have expiration dates. It's important to regularly check these dates and replace any items that have expired to ensure their effectiveness.

2. Keep the kit clean: A first aid kit should be kept in a clean and dry place to prevent contamination of the supplies. Regularly wipe down the outside of the kit and replace any items that have become soiled or damaged.

3. Refill used items: If you use any items from your first aid kit, be sure to replace them as soon as possible. This will ensure that your kit is always fully stocked and ready to use.

4. Consider your specific needs: A first aid kit should be tailored to your specific needs and activities. If you have any allergies or medical conditions, make sure to include necessary medication or supplies in your kit.

5. Keep a list of contents: It's a good idea to keep a list of the items in your first aid kit and their quantities. This will help you keep track of what needs to be restocked and can be helpful in emergencies when others may need to use the kit.

6. Replace old or damaged items: Regularly inspect your first aid kit for any items that may have become damaged or unusable. This can include items that have been exposed to extreme temperatures, liquids, or have expired.

7. Consider including additional items: Depending on your specific needs and activities, you may want to consider including additional items in your first aid kit. This can include items such as a CPR face shield, a first aid manual, or a tourniquet.

8. Store it in a visible and easily accessible location: In case of an emergency, it's important to have your first aid kit in a visible and easily accessible location. Make sure everyone in your household or workplace knows where the kit is located.

9. Keep track of any medications: If your first aid kit includes any medications, make sure to keep track of when they were opened and when they expire. It may be helpful to include this information on your list of contents.

10. Don't overstock your kit: While it's important to have a well-stocked first aid kit, it's also important not to overstock it. Make sure you have enough supplies for minor injuries and emergencies, but avoid including excessive amounts of items.

By following these tips for maintaining your first aid kit, you can ensure that it is ready for use in any situation. Remember to regularly check and restock your kit to keep yourself and others safe.

Educating Others on First Aid

Knowing how to administer first aid is a valuable skill that can save lives in the event of an emergency.

However, it's not just enough for an individual to have this knowledge – it's also important to educate others on the basics of first aid.

Here are some tips for educating others on first aid:

1. Lead by example: The best way to educate others on first aid is to lead by example. Practice proper first aid techniques in your daily life and encourage others to do the same. This will make the information more tangible and encourage others to take it seriously.

2. Use hands-on training: The best way to learn first aid is through hands-on training. If possible, organize or attend a first aid training course where participants can learn and practice techniques in a controlled environment. This will help build confidence and understanding of the skills.

3. Share resources: There are many resources available that can help educate others on first aid, such as books, videos, and online tutorials. Share these resources with friends, family, and coworkers to help them learn more about the basics of first aid.

4. Identify common scenarios: By identifying common scenarios where first aid may be needed, you can better prepare others for potential emergencies. For example, in the workplace, common scenarios may include burns, cuts, or sprains.

5. Teach the basics: It's important not to overwhelm others with too much information. Focus on teaching the basics of first aid, such as how to assess a situation, stop bleeding, and perform CPR. These skills can be used in a variety of situations and are easy to remember.

6. Use clear and simple language: When educating others on first aid, it's important to use clear and simple language. Avoid using medical jargon or technical terms that may confuse or intimidate others. This will make the information more understandable and relatable.

7. Encourage questions: Leave time for questions and make sure to address any uncertainties or concerns that others may have. This will help reinforce the information and provide a better understanding of the skills.

8. Practice regularly: Just like with any other skill, practicing regularly is key to retaining knowledge and improving proficiency. Encourage others to practice first aid techniques regularly and offer opportunities for hands-on practice if possible.

9. Offer refresher courses: As time goes by, it's easy for people to forget certain first aid skills. Consider offering refresher courses to remind others of the basics and any updates or changes in techniques.

10. Make it fun: Lastly, make the learning experience fun by incorporating games or activities that can help reinforce the information. This will make the process of learning first aid more enjoyable and engaging for others.

By educating others on how to administer first aid, you can help create a safer environment for everyone. Remember to lead by example, use hands-on training, and make the learning experience enjoyable.

Together, we can all be prepared for potential emergencies and stay safe.

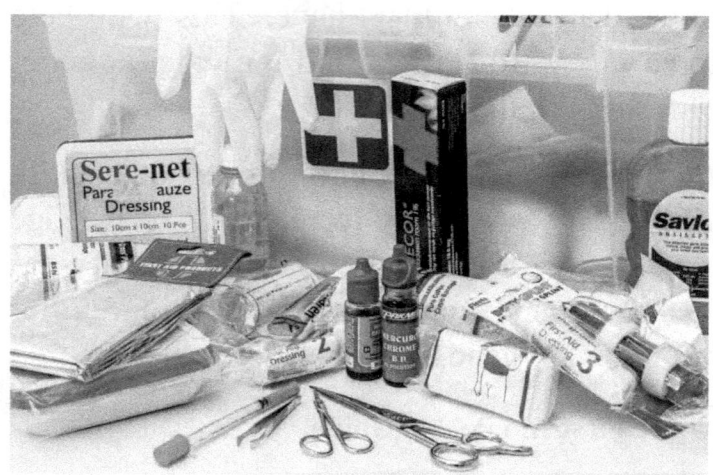

CHAPTER 9

Conclusion

Review

I recently had the opportunity to read the Basic First Aid Pocket Guide, and I must say, it is a must-have for anyone who wants to be prepared for emergencies. This compact guide is packed with essential information on how to handle a wide range of injuries or medical situations, making it a valuable resource for both experienced first aiders and those who have never received any formal training.

One of the things I appreciated most about this guide is its straightforward and concise approach. It is written in clear, easy-to-understand language, making it accessible to readers of all levels. The step-by-step instructions and accompanying illustrations make it even easier to follow and remember the correct procedures for each situation. I also appreciate that the guide covers a wide range of topics, from cuts and bruises to more serious situations like choking, cardiac arrest, and even snake bites.

Another aspect that makes this guide stand out is its portability. The pocket-size design makes it easy to carry with you at all times, whether you're going on a camping trip, a family vacation, or simply out for a walk. This means that you'll always have quick access to potentially life-saving information in case of an emergency.

In addition to its practicality and usefulness, I also found the Basic First Aid Pocket Guide to be well-organized and visually appealing. The information is presented in a logical and easy-to-navigate manner, with clear chapter divisions and bullet points for key takeaways. The illustrations are also well-drawn and provide an excellent visual aid to complement the written instructions.

Furthermore, I appreciate that the guide includes valuable tips on how to be prepared for emergencies, such as putting together a first aid kit and knowing important contact numbers. These extra details enhance the overall usefulness of the guide and demonstrate the author's commitment to providing comprehensive information.

If I had to suggest one improvement for the guide, it would be to include a section on providing first aid in emergency situations involving children.

While many of the techniques and procedures can apply to both adults and children, I believe having specific instructions for pediatric first aid would be beneficial.

Overall, I highly recommend the Basic First Aid Pocket Guide to anyone looking to be more prepared for emergencies. Its easy-to-understand instructions, comprehensive coverage, and compact design make it an essential resource to have on hand at all times. Whether you're a parent, a sports coach, or simply someone who wants to be able to help in case of an emergency, this guide has something of value for everyone.

Importance of Being Prepared

Being prepared is crucial when it comes to any emergency situation. This statement holds especially true when it comes to first aid situations. Accidents and emergencies can happen at any time, and having the right knowledge and tools at hand can make all the difference between life and death. This is where the Basic First Aid Pocket Guide comes in, making it an essential resource for being prepared in case of an emergency.

One of the most significant benefits of the basic first aid pocket guide is its portability. Its compact size allows you to carry it with you at all times, ensuring that you have access to life-saving information wherever you go.

In an emergency, every second counts, and having the guide readily available can mean the difference between providing immediate assistance and waiting for help to arrive.

Moreover, the guide provides clear and concise instructions on how to handle a range of injuries and emergencies. This is especially important for individuals who have not received any formal first aid training. The step-by-step procedures and accompanying illustrations make it easy to follow and remember, even in high-stress situations. Knowing what to do in an emergency can give you confidence and help you remain calm, which is crucial for providing effective first aid.

Another important aspect of being prepared is having the necessary tools and supplies on hand. The Basic First Aid Pocket Guide not only provides essential instructions but also includes tips on how to build a first aid kit and what to include in it.

This valuable information ensures that you have the necessary tools to administer first aid in case of an emergency.

Moreover, being prepared with first aid knowledge and resources can be beneficial in everyday situations as well. It can help you respond to minor injuries or illnesses encountered in daily life, such as cuts, burns, or food poisoning. This not only saves you time and money but also prevents potential medical complications.

In conclusion, the Basic First Aid Pocket Guide is more than just a first aid manual – it is a valuable resource for being prepared in case of any emergency. Its compact size, comprehensive coverage, and practical tips make it an essential item to have on hand at all times. By being prepared, you can not only potentially save a life but also increase your confidence and ability to handle any unexpected situation with ease.

Final Thoughts.

In conclusion, the Basic First Aid Pocket Guide is an excellent resource for anyone looking to be more prepared in case of an emergency. Its compact size, clear instructions, and comprehensive coverage make it an essential item to have on hand at all times. Whether you are a seasoned first aider or someone with no formal training, this guide provides valuable knowledge and tips on how to handle a variety of injuries and medical situations. Additionally, its portability and practicality make it a valuable resource for everyday situations as well. By having the Basic First Aid Pocket Guide, you can have peace of mind knowing that you are prepared to handle any emergency that comes your way. I highly recommend this guide to anyone who wants to be more equipped in case of an emergency. After all, being prepared is the first step towards being able to provide effective and potentially life-saving first aid.

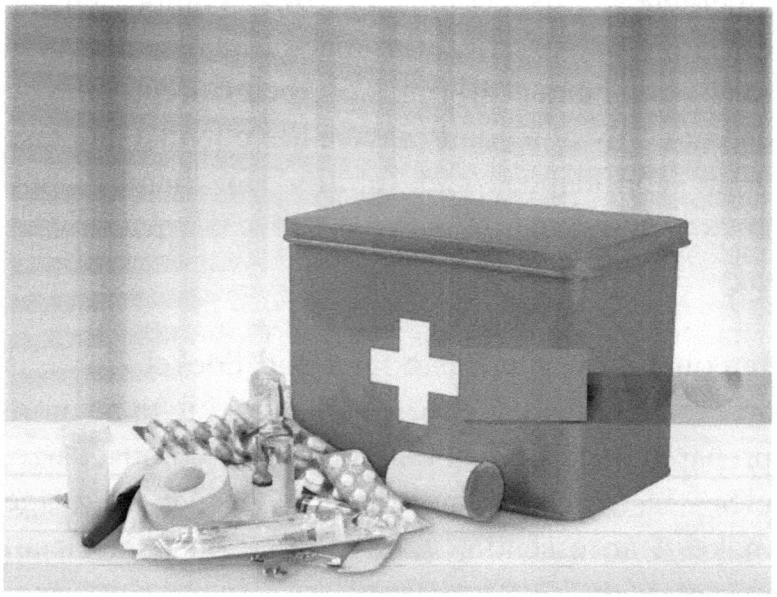

CHAPTER 10 BONUS
Some sample workout plans for beginners

1. Monday:

- 5-minute warm-up: Jog in place, do jumping jacks or skip rope

- 3 sets of 10 reps bodyweight squats

- 3 sets of 10 reps push-ups

- 3 sets of 10 reps walking lunges (5 each leg)

- 3 sets of 10 reps bench dips

- 3 sets of 10 reps wall sits

- 5-minute cool down: Stretching

2. Tuesday:

- 5-minute warm-up: Jog in place, do jumping jacks or skip rope

- 3 sets of 10 reps dumbbell bicep curls

- 3 sets of 10 reps dumbbell shoulder press

- 3 sets of 10 reps dumbbell upright rows

- Dumbbell upright rows, three sets of ten reps

- 3 sets of 10 reps dumbbell lateral raises

- 5-minute cool down: Stretching

3. Wednesday:

- 5-minute warm-up: Jog in place, do jumping jacks or skip rope

- 3 sets of 10 reps bodyweight deadlifts

- 3 sets of 10 reps stability ball leg curls

- 3 sets of 10 reps glute bridges

- Three sets of ten glute bridge reps

- 3 sets of 10 reps bicycle crunches

- 5-minute cool down: Stretching

4. Thursday:

- 5-minute warm-up: Jog in place, do jumping jacks or skip rope

- 3 sets of 10 reps dumbbell bench press

- 3 sets of 10 reps dumbbell rows

- Dumbbell rows for three sets of ten reps

- Dumbbell pullovers, three sets of ten repetitions

- 3 sets of 10 reps lat pulldowns

- 5-minute cool down: Stretching

5. Friday:

- 5-minute warm-up: Jog in place, do jumping jacks or skip rope

- 3 sets of 10 reps bodyweight squats to calf raises

- 3 sets of 10 reps mountain climbers

- 3 sets of 10 reps burpees

- 3 sets of 10 reps plank hold for 1 minute

- 3 sets of 10 reps Russian twists

- 5-minute cool down: Stretching

6. Saturday:

- 5-minute warm-up: Jog in place, do jumping jacks or skip rope

- 3 sets of 10 reps dumbbell lunges (5 each leg)

- 3 sets of 10 reps dumbbell step-ups

- 3 sets of 10 reps dumbbell Romanian deadlifts

- 3 sets of 10 reps kneeling push-ups

- 3 sets of 10 reps dumbbell lateral lunges (5 each leg)

- 5-minute cool down: Stretching

7. Sunday:

- Rest day or light cardio such as walking or swimming for 30 minutes.

8. Monday:

- 5-minute warm-up: Jog in place, do jumping jacks or skip rope

- 3 sets of 10 reps dumbbell chest press

- Dumbbell chest press, three sets of ten reps

- 3 sets of 10 reps dumbbell incline press

- 3 sets of 10 reps dumbbell front raises

- Ten reps of three sets of tricep dips

- 5-minute cool down: Stretching

9. Tuesday:

- 5-minute warm-up: Jog in place, do jumping jacks or skip rope

- 3 sets of 10 reps bodyweight squats to overhead press

- 3 sets of 10 reps jump squats

- 3 sets of 10 reps high knees

- 3 sets of 10 reps sumo squats

- 3 sets of 10 reps bicycle crunches

- 5-minute cool down: Stretching

10. Wednesday:

- 5-minute warm-up: Jog in place, do jumping jacks or skip rope

- 3 sets of 10 reps dumbbell hammer curls

- 3 sets of 10 reps dumbbell bent-over rows

- 3 sets of 10 reps dumbbell front squats

- 3 sets of 10 reps dumbbell shoulder raises

- Ten reps of three sets of tricep kickbacks

- 5-minute cool down: Stretching

11. Thursday:

- 5-minute warm-up: Jog in place, do jumping jacks or skip rope

- 3 sets of 10 reps walking lunges with dumbbells (5 each leg)

- 3 sets of 10 reps side lunges with dumbbells (5 each leg)

- 3 sets of 10 reps reverse lunges with dumbbells (5 each leg)

- Dumbbell calf lifts, three sets of ten reps

- 3 sets of 10 reps Russian twists

- 5-minute cool down: Stretching

12. Friday:

- 5-minute warm-up: Jog in place, do jumping jacks or skip rope

- 3 sets of 10 reps dumbbell chest flyes

- 3 sets of 10 reps dumbbell reverse flyes

- 3 sets of 10 reps dumbbell chest press with a twist

- 3 sets of 10 reps dumbbell bent-over rear delt raises

- 3 sets of 10 reps tricep overhead extensions

- 5-minute cool down: Stretching

13. Saturday:

- 5-minute warm-up: Jog in place, do jumping jacks or skip rope

- 3 sets of 10 reps goblet squats

- 3 sets of 10 reps Romanian deadlifts with dumbbells

- Three sets of ten donkey kick reps

- Three sets of ten fire hydrant repetitions

- 3 sets of 10 reps plank with shoulder taps

- 5-minute cool down: Stretching

14. Sunday:

- Rest day or light cardio such as walking or swimming for 30 minutes.

15. Monday:

- 5-minute warm-up: Jog in place, do jumping jacks or skip rope

- 3 sets of 10 reps bodyweight squats to jump squats

- 3 sets of 10 reps push-ups to rows (using dumbbells)

- 3 sets of 10 reps side plank dips

- 3 sets of 10 reps bicycle crunches

- 3 sets of 10 reps tricep dips with one leg lifted

- 5-minute cool down: Stretching

16. Tuesday:

- 5-minute warm-up: Jog in place, do jumping jacks or skip rope

- 3 sets of 10 reps dumbbell front raise to lateral raise

- 3 sets of 10 reps dumbbell shoulder press to front raises

- 3 sets of 10 reps dumbbell upright rows to lateral raises

- 3 sets of 10 reps dumbbell bicep curl to shoulder press

- 3 sets of 10 reps tricep skull crushers

- 5-minute cool down: Stretching

17. Wednesday:

- 5-minute warm-up: Jog in place, do jumping jacks or skip rope

- 3 sets of 10 reps jumping lunges (5 each leg)

- 3 sets of 10 reps plyometric push-ups

- Tuck leaps, three sets of ten reps

- Three sets of ten box jump reps

- 3 sets of 10 reps plank with shoulder taps and hip dips

- 5-minute cool down: Stretching

18. Thursday:

- 5-minute warm-up: Jog in place, do jumping jacks or skip rope

- 3 sets of 10 reps dumbbell chest flyes on stability ball

- 3 sets of 10 reps dumbbell pullovers on stability ball

- 3 sets of 10 reps tricep dips on stability ball

- 3 sets of 10 reps single legged bridges on stability ball

- 3 sets of 10 reps bicycle crunches on stability ball

- 5-minute cool down: Stretching

19. Friday:

- 5-minute warm-up: Jog in place, do jumping jacks or skip rope

- 3 sets of 10 reps single arm dumbbell rows

- 3 sets of 10 reps dumbbell renegade rows

- 3 sets of 10 reps seated dumbbell shoulder press

- 3 sets of 10 reps bicep curls with resistance bands

- 3 sets of 10 reps tricep kickbacks with resistance bands

- 5-minute cool down: Stretching

20. Saturday:

- 5-minute warm-up: Jog in place, do jumping jacks or skip rope

- 3 sets of 10 reps goblet squats to calf raises
- 3 sets of 10 reps dumbbell plie squats
- 3 sets of 10 reps sumo deadlifts with dumbbells
- 3 sets of 10 reps dumbbell thrusters
- 3 sets of 10 reps mountain climbers
- 5-minute cool down: Stretching

www.ingramcontent.com/pod-product-compliance
Lightning Source LLC
Chambersburg PA
CBHW050310230526
45471CB00005B/2115